The Best Cookbook for Pregnant Women

Discover 35 Recipes Guaranteed to help you and your Baby stay Healthy

By

Heston Brown

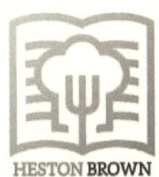

HESTON BROWN

Copyright 2019 Heston Brown

Thank you so much for buying my book! I want to give you a special gift!

Receive a special gift as a thank you for buying my book. Now you will be able to benefit from free and discounted book offers that are sent directly to your inbox every week.

To subscribe simply fill in the box below with your details and start reaping the rewards! A new deal will arrive every day and reminders will be sent so you never miss out. Fill in the box below to subscribe and get started!

https://heston-brown.getresponsepages.com

Subscribe
to our
newsletter

Your Email

Table of Contents

Recipe 1: The Vegetable Omelet

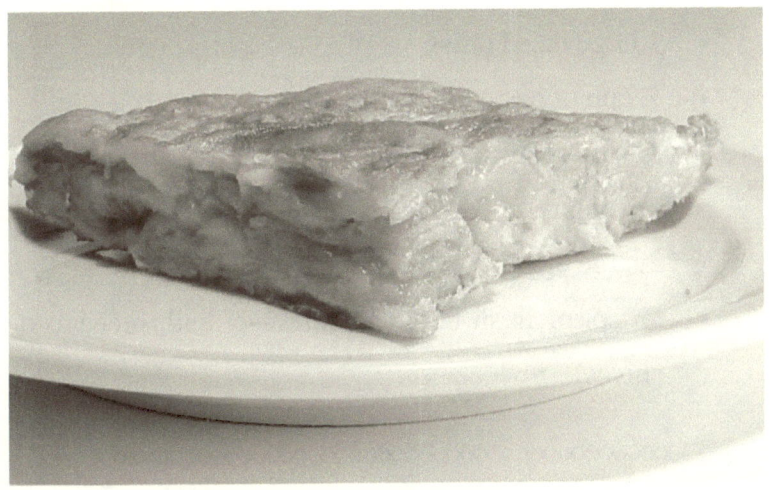

This recipe is ideal for the vegetarian mom.

Cooking Time: 20 minutes

Serving Size: 2

List of List of Ingredients:

- 2 large sliced or crushed tomatoes,
- 1 large diced onion,
- ½ cup of pasteurized goat cheese,
- A cup of a mix of broccoli, kale, bell pepper, and asparagus
- 2 large eggs.
- ½ tsp. of fresh herb (for instance; bail, oregano or chives).

xxxxxxxxxxxxxxxxxxxxxxxxxxxxxxxxxxxxxxxxxxx

Instructions:

Make omelet with the mi of your veggies and eggs, then add the herb for some flavour and serve immediately.

Recipe 2: Fast Egg-Muffin (Breakfast)

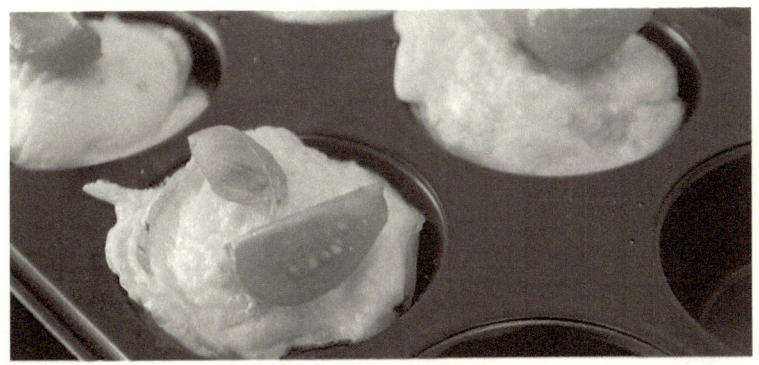

The recipe is convenient and each muffin provides about 96 calories, plus 6g of fat, and 1g of carb.

Cooking Time: 45 minutes

Serving Size: 6

List of Ingredients:

- 5-6 eggs,
- 6 slices of turkey,
- 1/2 cup of chopped and sliced spinach,
- 2-3 Tbsp. of red pepper,
- a scoop of mozzarella cheese,
- Optional tsp. of fresh basil
- 2 small chopped and sliced red onions, and
- A tsp. of salt and pepper.

xxxxxxxxxxxxxxxxxxxxxxxxxxxxxxxxxxxxxxxxxxx

Instructions:

Pre-heat the oven to about 350 degrees, and then prepare the spinach, red pepper and basil before grating the cheese. Spray a non-sticking muffin tin with some olive oil, and gently drape the turkey inside one of the muffin cups, and then crack an egg inside the cup. Add all the ingredients, and then put the muffin tin inside the oven and cook for about 15 minutes. Enjoy the muffins.

Recipe 3: The Chicken and Tomato Pasta, Served with Snow Peas

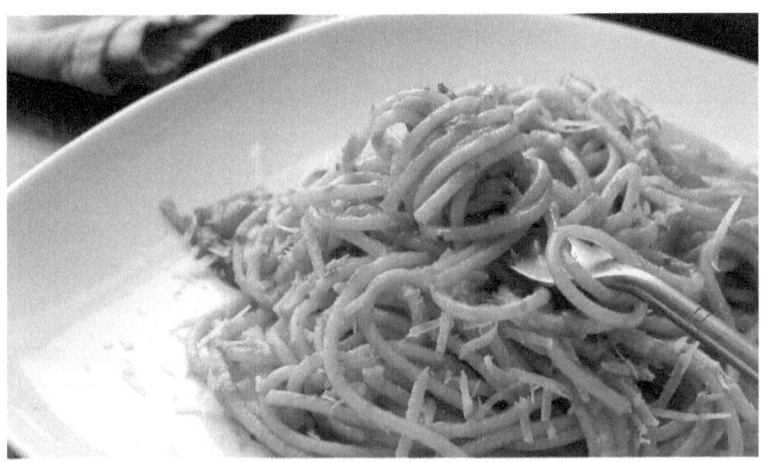

This is a low-calorie nutritious chicken meal every month will love to relish.

Cooking Time: 1-2 hour

Serving Size: 1-2

List of List of Ingredients:

- 100g of trimmed and halved snow peas,
- About 250g of dried penne pasta,
- 400-500g of chicken breast fillet,
- A tsp. of olive oil, and
- 1 standard bottle or 500g of Tomato and Basil pasta sauce.

xxxxxxxxxxxxxxxxxxxxxxxxxxxxxxxxxxxxxxxxxxxxx

Instructions:

In large saucepan containing boiling water, simply cook the pasta, then add the snow peas and after cooking, drain. Pre-heat a medium or large frying pan over medium heat, before brushing the chicken with olive oil. Season the chicken with some salt and pepper before cooking each side of the chicken for about 4 minutes. Slice the chicken before adding the pasta mix, toss and divide in bowls before serving.

Recipe 4: The Turkey Burger

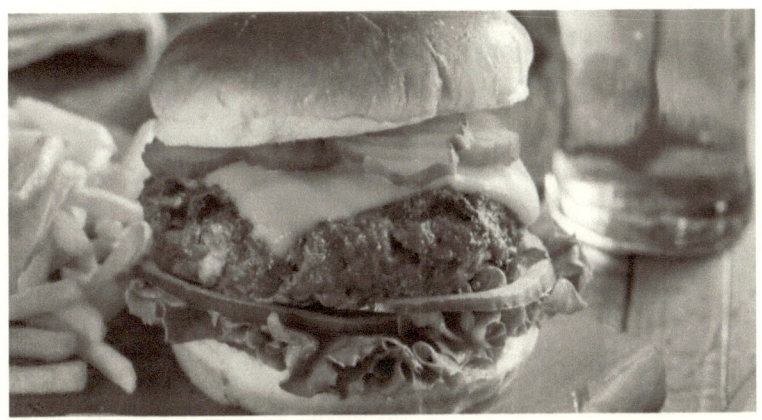

Do you feel like snacking? Just make yourself a quick, delicious burger made up of turkey.

Preparation: about 1 hour

Serving Size: 1-2

List of Ingredients:

- 2 moderate portions of turkey breasts,
- Collard green wrap,
- Tomatoes,
- 1 large onion,
- A tsp. of grape-seed oil,

xxxxxxxxxxxxxxxxxxxxxxxxxxxxxxxxxxxxxxxxxxxxx

Instructions:

Mix the ingredients and then add into a collard, then add salsa and tomatoes. Top up with avocado and onion before coating with grape seed oil. Season the burger before baking.

Recipe 5: Grilled Vegetables Served with Snapper

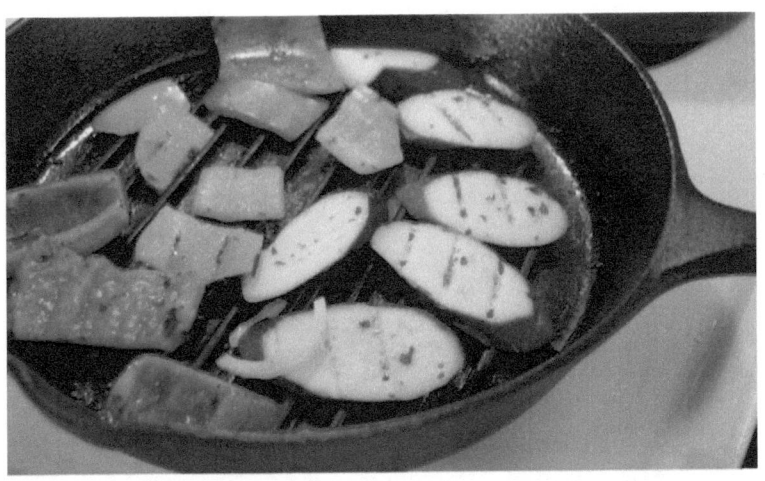

This Is an Inspiring and Very Nutritious Meal For A Growing Pregnancy.

Cooking Time: 30 minutes

Serving Size: 2-4

List of Ingredients:

- 2 large Japanese egg plants,
- 3-4 Zucchinis,
- 2 large potatoes,
- 1 large red onion
- 1 capsicum,
- 1/3 cup of olive oil,
- 8 sprigs thyme,
- 4 snapper skin fillets,
- A quarter bunch of basil,
- 2 Tbsp. of vinegar,
- 80g of pitted kalamata olives.

xxxxxxxxxxxxxxxxxxxxxxxxxxxxxxxxxxxxxxxxxxxx

Instructions:

Pre-heat a medium to large size barbecue to medium-high heat, then cut the eggplant, tomato and zucchinis, into halves while the onion is cut into 6 wedges. Cut the capsicum and add the vegetables in a bowl. Drizzle with oil, then add your pepper, salt and thyme sprigs inside the bowl and mix. Cook all vegetables until they are about to char and transfer them unto a cutting board. Halve the zucchini and egg plants and mix with the rest of the vegetables in a bowl before drizzling the vinegar and oil. Split the veggies over the basil leaves, toss and combine before topping it with the prepared fish filets.

Recipe 6: The Burrito Bowl

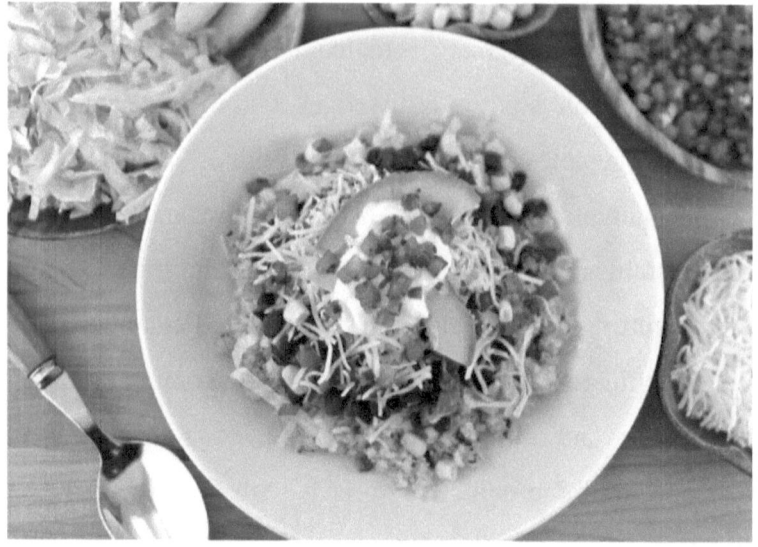

This is a perfect breakfast or dinner recipe with a great taste.

Cooking Time: 40 minutes

Serving Size: 1-2

List of Ingredients:

- A cup of brown rice,
- 2 diced and roasted red pepper,
- ½ cup of beans,
- 1-2 sliced lean meat,
- 1-2 roasted tomatoes,
- 1 avocado,
- Juice of one lemon

xxxxxxxxxxxxxxxxxxxxxxxxxxxxxxxxxxxxxxxxxxx

Instructions:

Cook the brown rice for about 20 minutes, then add your ingredients, including the pepper, beans, lean meat, tomatoes, and then top with the avocado and lemon juice.

Recipe 7: Creamy Chicken Served with Sun-Dried Tomato Pasta

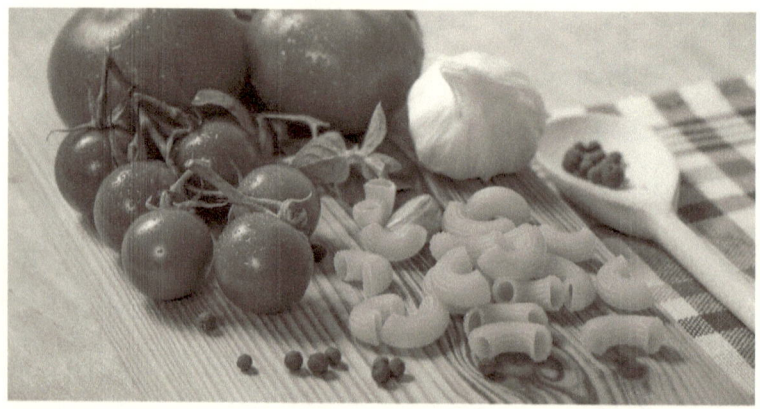

This is an easy pasta with chicken recipe you can consider for lunch. It is simply delicious in addition to offering essential Protein, fat, and Vitamins.

Cooking Time: 35 minutes

Serving Size: 4-7

List of List of Ingredients:

- ½ portion of chicken breast,
- 1 large peeled banana,
- 1 Tbsp. of olive oil,
- 1 cup of boiling water,
- ½ Tbsp. of pepper and salt.

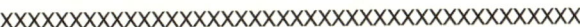

Instructions:

Pre-heat the oven until 350 degrees. First, prepare your pasta by bringing it to boil over high heat, and allow to cook for about 5 minutes or more. Prepare your chicken (preferably chicken breast, because it contains much less fat). Slice your banana in a food processor until it becomes marshy. Bake the chicken for about 20 minutes, while hot, spread the marshy banana on its surface and serve immediately.

Recipe 8: The South-Western Scramble

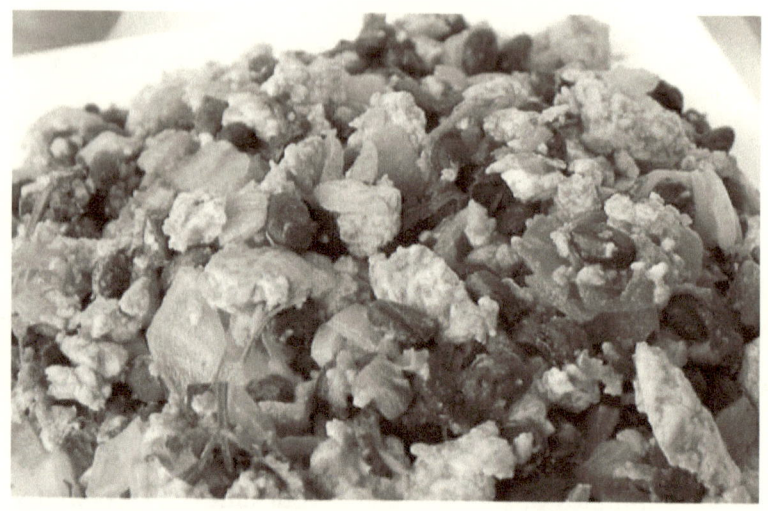

Another nutritious scramble to start your day.

Cooking Time: 15 minutes

Serving Size: 1

List of Ingredients:

- Hatch chiles,
- 2 large eggs,
- 1 large onion,
- a moderate size shredded chicken,
- 1 large avocado.

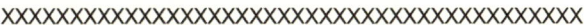

Instructions:

Scramble the mix together over medium heat, and simmer for extra few minutes before serving.

Recipe 9: Barbecue Chili, Served with Sesame Beef and Red Cabbage Slaw

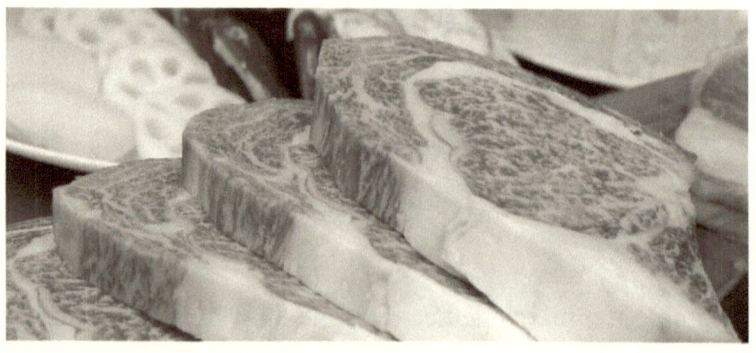

A perfect source of protein and healthy fat for you and the baby.

Cooking Time: 20

Serving Size: 8

List of Ingredients:

- 1-2 tsp. of sesame seeds,
- 2 peeled garlic cloves,
- ¼ cup of soil sauce,
- 2 tsp. of Sambal oelek,
- 2 tsp. of caster sugar,
- ¼ cup of white vinegar,
- 1-2 Tbsp. of vegetable oil,
- 3 boneless steaks of sirloin (these must by fat-trimmed and thinly sliced),
- ¼ thinly sliced cabbage,
- 2 trimmed green onions,
- 2 cut red radishes,
- Medium grain steamed rice (1-2 cups should be enough).

xxxxxxxxxxxxxxxxxxxxxxxxxxxxxxxxxxxxxxxxxxxx

Instructions:

Pre-heat your barbecue on high heat, before placing the sesame seeds on a frying pan. Toast the seeds for about 1 minute, gently transfer the sesame seed into the mortar and add the garlic before pounding the mix. Add other ingredients and stir again. Place the beef in a medium size bowl, and stir them in a quarter of the sesame mixture, cover and set aside. Combine the cabbage, radish, green onions, and the remaining sesame dressing. Cook the beef for about 2-3 minutes, then toss them in the other mix until perfectly cooked together. Serve immediately.

Recipe 10: The Cookie Dough Cereal Meal

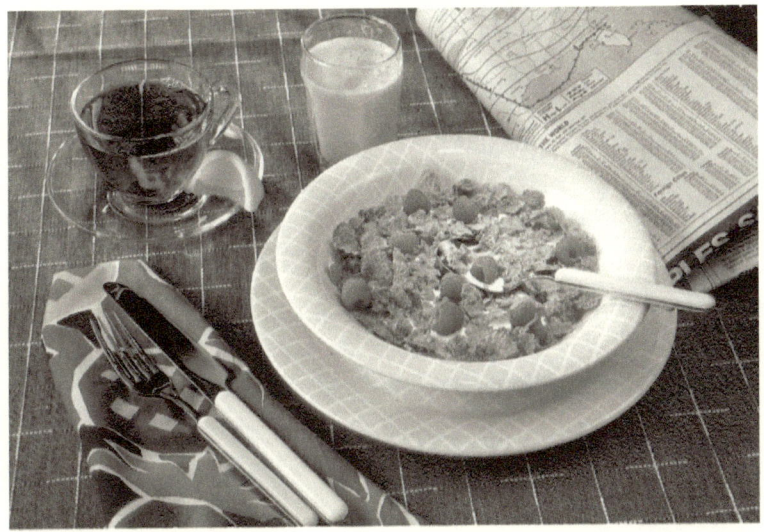

Whole cereal is good for both mother and baby, therefore, take some time to enjoy this delicacy.

Cooking Time: 15-25 minutes

Serving Size: 1-2

List of List of Ingredients:

- ½ cup of organic rolled oats,
- 2 tsp. of but butter,
- 1 tsp. of raw honey,
- 1 tsp. of unsweetened cocoa powder,
- ½ cup of non-fat milk.

xxxxxxxxxxxxxxxxxxxxxxxxxxxxxxxxxxxxxxxxxxxx

Instructions:

Mix all the ingredients until the mix becomes crumbly, then add the mix before serving.

Recipe 11: Spiced Salmon Served with Broccolini and Asparagus

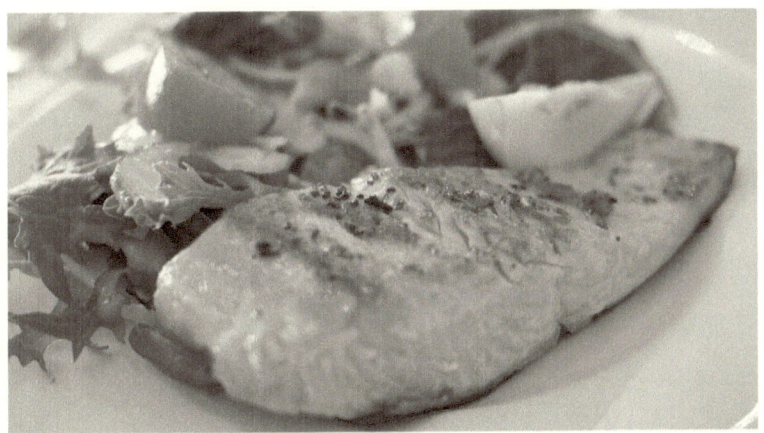

Salmon provides healthy omega 3 fats which is healthy to regulate your cholesterol. Combine this with the benefits inside asparagus and broccolini, then you have a perfect dinner.

Cooking Time: 1 hour

Serving Size: 2-4

List of Ingredients:

- 4 pieces of boneless salmon fillets,
- A Tbsp. of five-spice (Chinese spice),
- ½ a cup of hoisin sauce,
- ½ a cup of peanut oil,
- 2 cloves of thinly sliced garlic,
- A thinly sliced large red onion,
- 3 slices of average ginger,
- A bunch of trimmed broccolini,
- A bunch of trimmed and halved asparagus,
- A bunch of baby spinach,
- 1 cup of basil leaves, and
- A tsp. of sesame oil.

xxxxxxxxxxxxxxxxxxxxxxxxxxxxxxxxxxxxxxxxxxx

Instructions:

Cut the fish into 3 (lengthwise), and place them in a large bowl before adding the spice and peanut oil. Season the mix with salt and pepper and toss. Heat a Tbsp. of oil in a pan, over a high heat and then add the fish before cooking for about 2 minutes. Transfer unto a plate, and then add the broccolini and asparagus before cooking spinach separately. Add the spinach after cooking for about 5 minutes, to the fish and serve immediately with boiled rice.

Recipe 12: The Delicious Breakfast Tacos

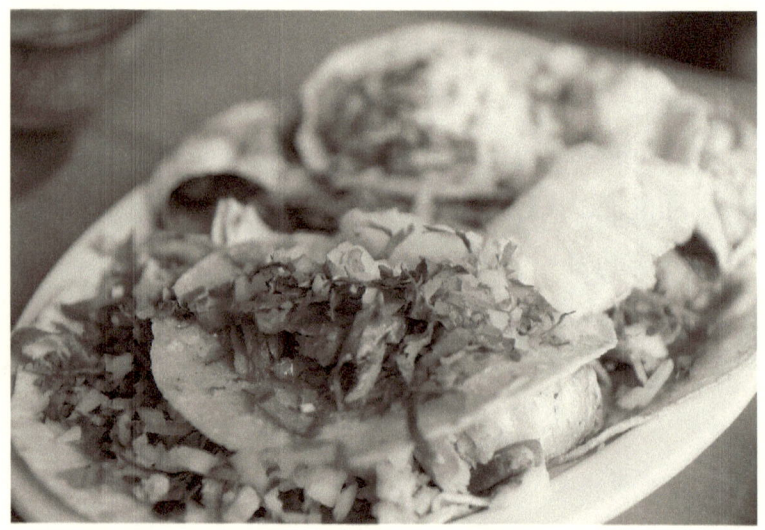

A perfect start to a new day for the expecting mom

Cooking Time: 40-45 minutes

Serving Size: 4-5

List of List of Ingredients:

- 3-4 large eggs,
- A cup of organic shredded cheese,
- 3 portions of lean meat,
- 3 cups of warm tortillas,
- Some sliced bell peppers.

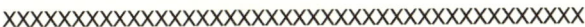

Instructions:

Scramble the eggs and add the lean meat, then sprinkle the cheese on top of the mix before serving in a warm tortilla that contains corn.

Recipe 13: Date with Carrot Puddings

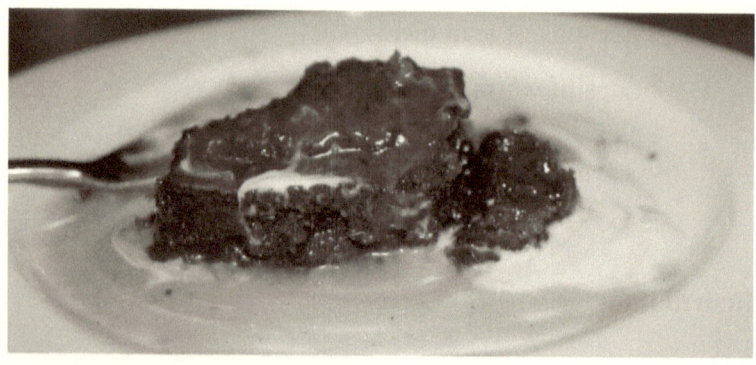

This is a perfect dinner recipe for any Pregnancy Cookbook.

Cooking Time: 30 minutes

Serving Size: 2-3

List of Ingredients:

- ½ cup of fresh, chopped dates,
- 2 tsp. of non-fat dairy spread,
- 1 Tbsp. of brown sugar,
- A medium to large size egg,
- A tsp. of vanilla essence,
- 1 large grated carrot,
- A tsp. of pure icing sugar.

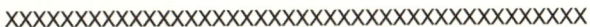

Instructions:

Pre-heat your oven to about 190 degrees, then grease some 4 (200mls) ramekins, and line the inner part of each with baking paper. Mix the dates inside half a cup of water, and heat over medium heat. Let the mix simmer for about 2 minutes and then set aside to cool. With the aid of an electric mixer, simply beat the sugar and spread until they are perfectly mixed. Add the egg and vanilla essence and mi perfectly. Stir in the carrot and date mix. Gently sift the flour over the date, and stir gently before using a spoon to pour it inside the ramekins, then place on the baking spray. Bake the mix for about 20 minutes, and let it stand for about 5 minutes before turning them in the serving plates. Serve immediately.

Recipe 14: The Sweet Potato Hash

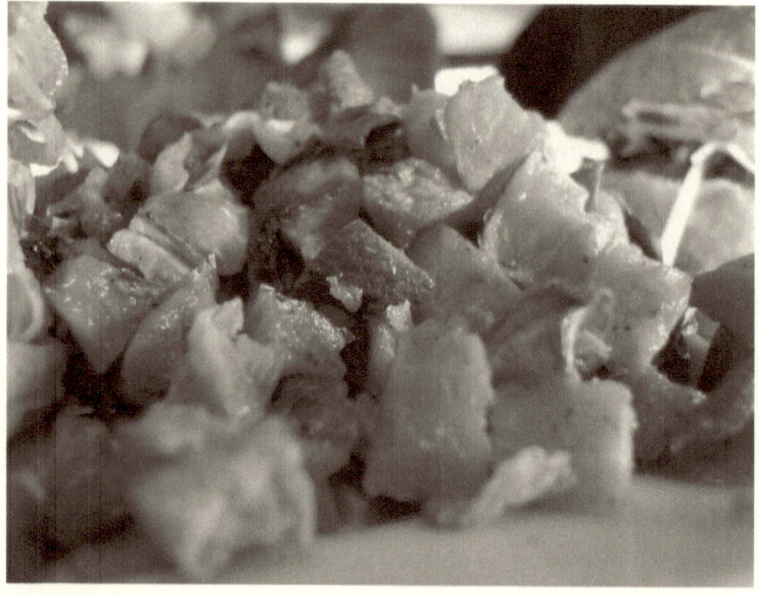

Enjoy the rejuvenating powers of sweet potato with this easy recipe.

Cooking Time: less than 45 minutes

Serving Size: 1

List of Ingredients:

- 1-2 eggs,
- 1 portion of lean meat or left-over turkey,
- Chopped veggies (any of your choice),
- 1 large sweet potato (diced).

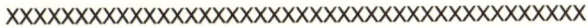

xxxxxxxxxxxxxxxxxxxxxxxxxxxxxxxxxxxxxxxxxxxx

Instructions:

Cook the scrambled eggs first, and then add the lean meat or sausage turkey, along with the chopped veggies and the sweet potato. Cook everything inside the skillet for about 10 minutes. Serve immediately.

Recipe 15: Barbecue Periperi Pork Served with Quick Guacamole

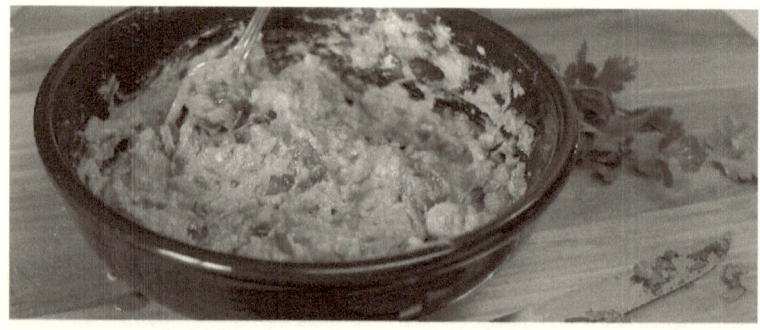

A sumptuous meal to give you energy and nutrients all day long.

Cooking Time: 30 minutes

Serving Size: 4

List of Ingredients:

- 3-4 pork cutlets, perfectly trimmed, and bones removed,
- ½ cup of periperi marmalade,
- 1 bunch of baby lettuce with leaves separated,
- A Tbsp. of olive oil,
- halve sliced lime.
- For the quick Guacamole, you need a flesh of 1 avocado
- juice extracted from half lime
- ¼ cup of chopped coriander leaves.

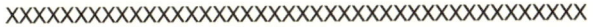

xxxxxxxxxxxxxxxxxxxxxxxxxxxxxxxxxxxxxxxxxx

Instructions:

With the aid of a meat mallet, simply beat the pork until it becomes slightly thicker, rub the marinade on it and let it stand for about 5 minutes. For the Guacamole, gently marsh the avocado with a fork, and then stir it in juice before stirring in the juice and coriander. Season the mi to your preferred taste, toss the entire mi in the bowl and then add half of the oil. Heat the remaining half of olive oil on a non-sticky fry pan and over medium heat. Cook the pork in the olive oil for about 5 minutes, and o not turn more than once. Remove the pan from heat after 5 minutes and cover the pork, serve immediately with the Guacamole and halved lime.

Recipe 16: Egg Muffins

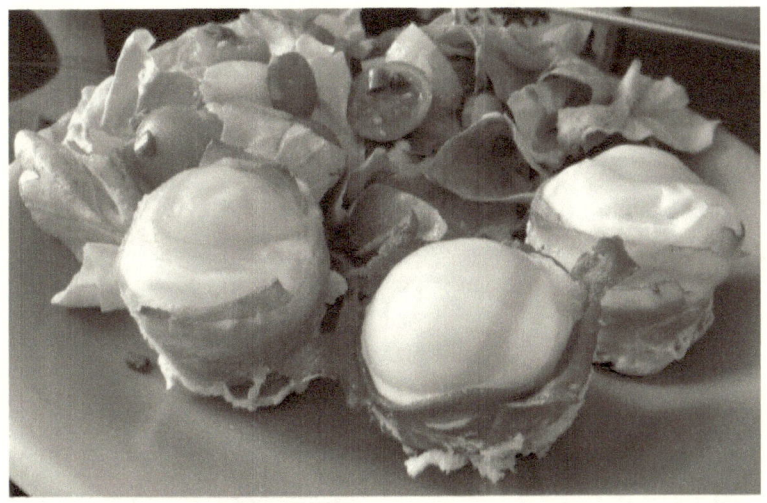

Great protein-rich recipe for breakfast or as snack for lunch.

Cooking Time: 20-30 minutes

Serving Size: 2-3

List of Ingredients:

- A handful of chopped vegetables (preferably, leafy green veggies)
- 1g of lean meat (this could be beef, chicken, lamb or turkey), and
- 2-3 medium to extra-large eggs.

xxxxxxxxxxxxxxxxxxxxxxxxxxxxxxxxxxxxxxxxxxxxxxx

Instructions:

Chopped the leafy veggies, and add them to the lean meat and pour the mix into a non-sticky muffin pan. Whisk the egg and pour it over the top of the meat and veggies, before baking the mi in the oven until about 350 degrees until it turns brown. You may increase the quantities of these recipes and prepare a large batch that can be re-heated when needed.

Recipe 17: The Whole Grain Fruit and Nut Muffins

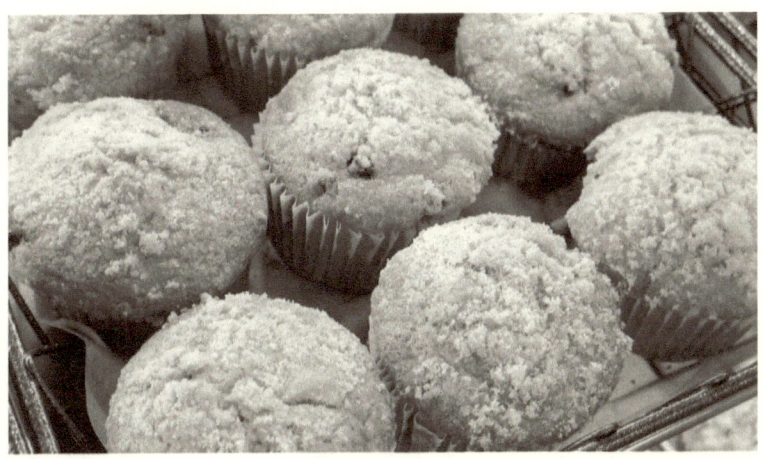

This recipe comes with great taste and texture, and it is the perfect one for those allergic to gluten in processed foods.

Cooking Time: 1 hour

Serving Size: 12 muffins

List of Ingredients:

- ¾ cup of gluten-free baking mix,
- ¾ cup of whole grain flour,
- 2 tsp. of baking powder,
- ½ tsp. of baking soda,
- ½ tsp. of salt,
- 2 medium-large eggs,
- ¾ cup of sugar,
- ¾ cup of low-fat butter milk,
- ½ tsp. of vanilla extract,
- 1 ½ cups of chopped fresh fruits, and
- 1 ½ cup of frozen berries.

xxxxxxxxxxxxxxxxxxxxxxxxxxxxxxxxxxxxxxxxxxxx

Instructions:

Step 1: pre-heat the oven to about 350 degrees, and coat your muffin cups with cooking spray.

Step2: whish the gluten-free mix, then whisk the egg, sugar, butter milk and vanilla in a separate bowl. Stir these in the mix and fold it in the fresh fruits and nuts.

Step 3: scoop the batter inside the muffin cups and bake for about 15 minutes. Cool immediately and serve.

Recipe 18: The Pb&J Oatmeal

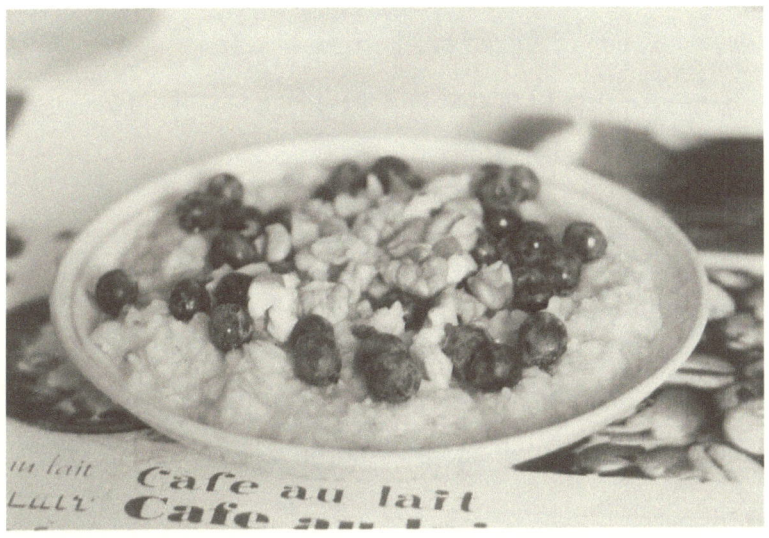

A perfect recipe for a quick meal. This is a nutritious meal with lots of fiber.

Cooking Time: 30 minutes

Serving Size: 1-2

List of Ingredients:

- ½ cup of organic rolled oats,
- ½ cup of frozen blueberries,
- A Tbsp. of peanut butter (this must contain no sugar, salt or oil).

xxxxxxxxxxxxxxxxxxxxxxxxxxxxxxxxxxxxxxxxxxxxxxx

Instructions:

Add the rolled oats, as directed, to the blueberries and then add the peanut butter and mix thoroughly before serving.

Recipe 19: Butter Nut, Banana and Chia Seeds Toast

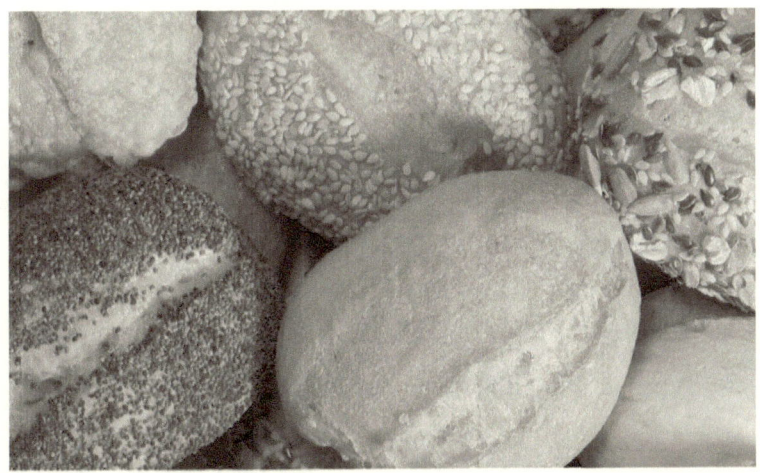

This recipe is packed with essential minerals and vitamins to get your day going. This recipe should take less than 40 minutes. This could be a perfect meal for dinner, when you don't require heavy meals.

Cooking Time: less than 40 minutes

Serving Size: 2-4

List of List of Ingredients:

- ½ sliced large banana,
- ½ tsp. of chia seeds
- 4 Tbsp. of nut butter
- 2 slice of 100% whole wheat bread

xxxxxxxxxxxxxxxxxxxxxxxxxxxxxxxxxxxxxxxxxx

Instructions:

Simply toast the bread and spread the nut butter at the top, add, the sliced banana at the top of the chia seed, toast and enjoy.

Recipe 20: The Low-Fat Creamy Pasta

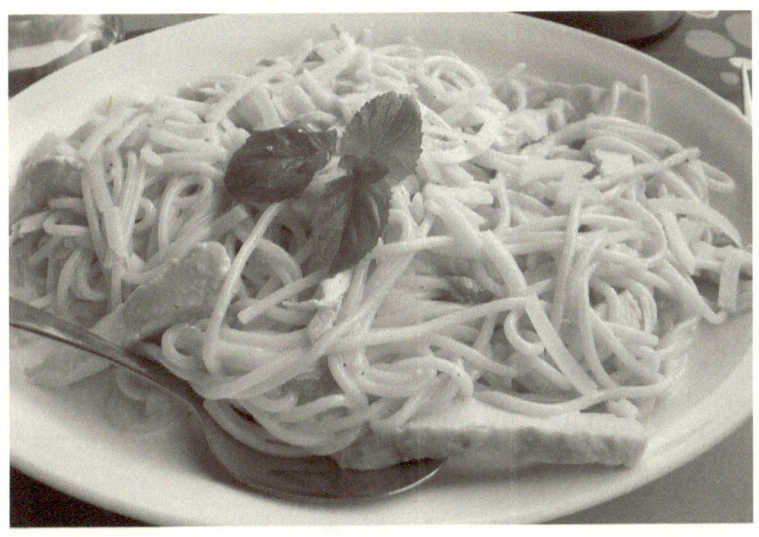

A perfect way to start your day.

Cooking Time: 24 minutes

Serving Size: 2

List of Ingredients:

- 150g of spaghetti pasta,
- 1 tsp. of olive oil,
- 2 chicken breast (fillet),
- A large brown, finely chopped onion,
- 2 thinly sliced garlic cloves,
- 2-3 moderate size cherry tomatoes,
- A can of light, and creamy evaporated milk,
- 2 tsp. of thyme leaves.
- 2 Tbsp. of chives (fresh),
- A cup of baby spinach,
- ½ cup of parmesan cheese.

xxxxxxxxxxxxxxxxxxxxxxxxxxxxxxxxxxxxxxxxxxx

Instructions:

Cook the spaghetti in a sauce pan inside a cup of water and over a medium heat. Drain the pasta and return the pan. Cover the cooked pasta to keep it warm, then heat half of the olive oil and cook the chicken inside for about 10 minutes. Add the onion and garlic until they become soft with the chicken. Add the tomatoes, thyme, evaporated milk, and baby spinach. Toss the mix and combine for about 3-5 minutes and remove from heat. Serve immediately.

Recipe 21: Macadamia Ricotta Served with Tomato Toast

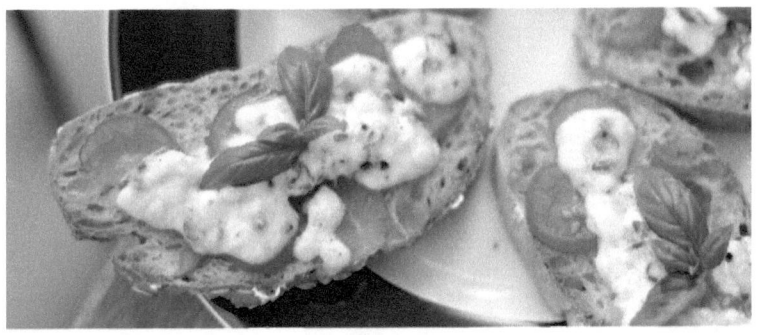

This is a good source of macro nutrients

Cooking Time: 1 hour

Serving Size: 2-6

List of Ingredients:

- a cup of soaked macadamia nuts,
- 1 ½ tsp. of nutritional yeast,
- 2 tsp. of apple cider vinegar,
- 1 ½ tsp. of lemon juice,
- 2 tsp. of white mellow miso taste,
- 2 garlic cloves,
- ½ a cup of filtered water, and
- ¼ tsp. of sea salt.

xxxxxxxxxxxxxxxxxxxxxxxxxxxxxxxxxxxxxxxxxxxx

Instructions:

Step 1: Rinse and drain the macadamia nuts and place in blender with the yeast and other ingredients (including water). Scrape the side of the blender and add a tsp. of water at a time when blending until you achieve a creamy consistency. Add the salt, vinegar and lemon sparingly for some taste, then transfer it to the refrigerator.

Step 2: remove the Macadamia ricotta from the fridge after 20 minutes and top your tasted bread with it before adding some extra salt and pepper for taste. Cut into slices and serve immediately

Recipe 22: The Minestrone Soups

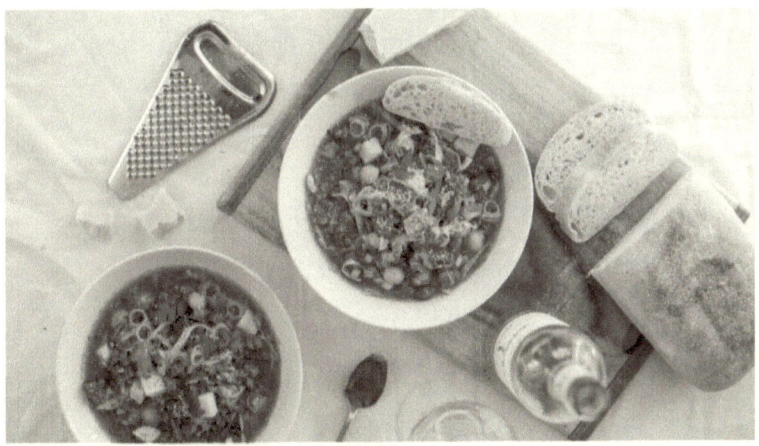

A delicious soup for dinner or lunch, and you can prepare enough to serve up to times. It takes about 50 minutes to prepare.

Cooking Time: 50 minutes

Serving Size: 2-3

List of Ingredients:

- 1 Tbsp. of cold-pressed rapeseed oil,
- 1 finely chopped medium or large onion,
- 2 big crushed clove garlic,
- 2 stalks of chopped celery,
- 2 medium chopped zucchini courgettes,
- 8 medium chopped carrots,
- 2 cups of chopped Spinach,
- Three 400g tins of chopped tomatoes,
- 150g of strand pasta,
- 5 pints of vegetable stock,
- 2 Tbsp. of tomato puree,
- freshly ground pepper with salt, and
- A handful of freshly chopped parsley.

xxxxxxxxxxxxxxxxxxxxxxxxxxxxxxxxxxxxxxxxxxx

Instructions:

cook the soup by sautéing the onion in garlic, inside the rapeseed oil until it becomes soft and translucent, add the celery and the courgette alongside the carrots and then cook for few minutes. Add your tomatoes, tomato puree, spinach, and vegetable stock, then mix very well before boiling. Reduce the heat and cover the mix gently to allow it simmer for about 15 minutes.

Add your pasta and then cook for extra 15 minutes, before seasoning (you can add fresh herbs if you want). Serve this soup immediately.

Recipe 23: Baked Salmon for The Expectant Mommy

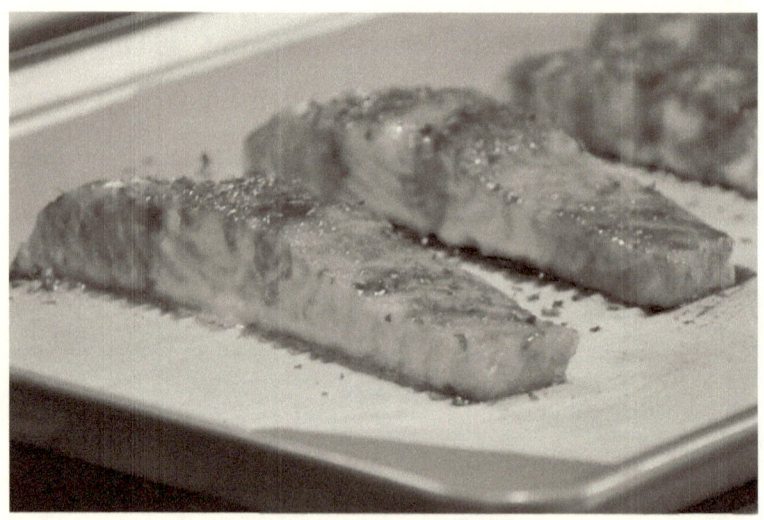

Salmon provides a very rich source of healthy Omega 3 fat, and you can serve this meal with a bowl of vegetable. Total calories for this recipe are about 353.

Cooking Time: 30 minutes

Serving Size: 1-2

List of Ingredients:

- 1 can of Salmon in tomato or chili sauce,
- 1 bowl of cooked vegetables (optional),
- 1 cup of non-sugary fruit juice prepared from the juice extractor or blender,
- ½ cup of boiling water, and
- 2 tsp. of olive oil.

xxxxxxxxxxxxxxxxxxxxxxxxxxxxxxxxxxxxxxxxxxxxx

Instructions:

Cook the vegetables (preferably spinach or broccoli) inside a ½ cup boiling water over medium to high heat, then turn on your oven and set the temperature at about 150 degrees. Then spray the baking pan with olive oil before pouring the salmon and then bake for about 5 minutes. Serve fresh and hot.

Recipe 24: Low Calorie Coffee Shakes (Breakfast)

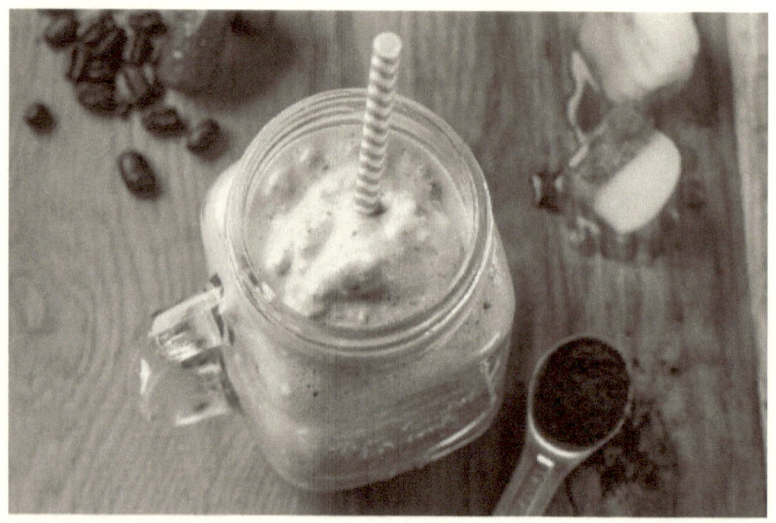

You need to be careful drinking coffee during pregnancy, therefore drink it sparingly.

Cooking Time: 25 minutes

Serving Size: 1-2

List of Ingredients:

- 1 scoop of Vanilla protein powder (with no sugar),
- A moderate shot of espresso or ½ tsp. of espresso,
- 1/4 cup of medium fat, Greek yoghurt,
- A Pinch of Stevia,
- A single pinch of Cinnamon, and
- 4 ice cubes.

xxxxxxxxxxxxxxxxxxxxxxxxxxxxxxxxxxxxxxxxxxx

Instructions:

Prepare your coffee, then add all the ingredients, including the protein powder inside the blender, and blend until perfectly smooth. Consume immediately.

Recipe 25: Sardine-Spinach and Tomato Soup (Dinner)

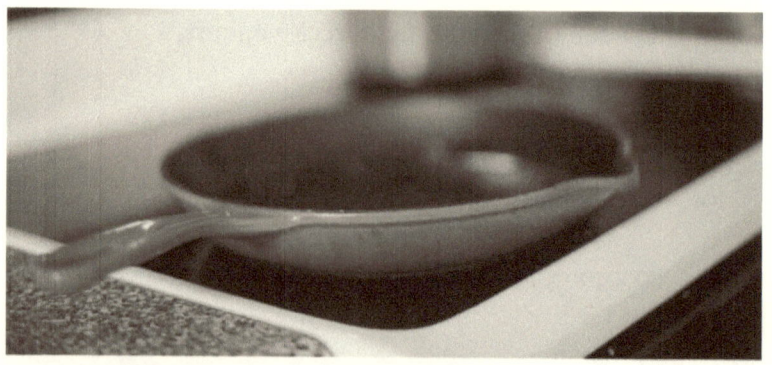

This is a perfect, delicious and nutritious soup you can enjoy at any period of the day but it is most suitable for dinners.

Cooking Time: less than 1 hour

Serving Size: 2-4

List of Ingredients:

- 2 Tbsp. of vegetable or corn oil,
- a Tbsp. of crushed garlic,
- a whole sliced onion,
- a large sliced tomato,
- 1 can of Spanish sardines inside tomato soup,
- 2-3 cups of vegetable broth,
- 1-2 cups of fresh baby spinach,
- A tsp. of salt and pepper, and
- A tsp. of black pepper powder.

xxxxxxxxxxxxxxxxxxxxxxxxxxxxxxxxxxxxxxxxxx

Instructions:

Put your vegetable or corn oil inside a medium size pot and prepare on a medium heat, sauté the garlic, tomato and onions and cook them for about 5 minutes until they become soft and tender. Add the sardines and mix very well to release the flavour, add the broth and let the mix boil before lowering the heat to medium. Add the spinach, pepper and salt, and serve while it's hot.

Childbirth and Pregnancy Nutrition

Easy smoothies and meals on the go, for busy pregnant mothers

Sometimes Childbirth and Pregnancy Nutrition can become tedious and all you want to do is grab something to drink. There are quite a number of healthy smoothies that will make your growing baby feel happy while getting enough nutrients for its health.

Recipe 26: Roasted Shrimps with Veggies

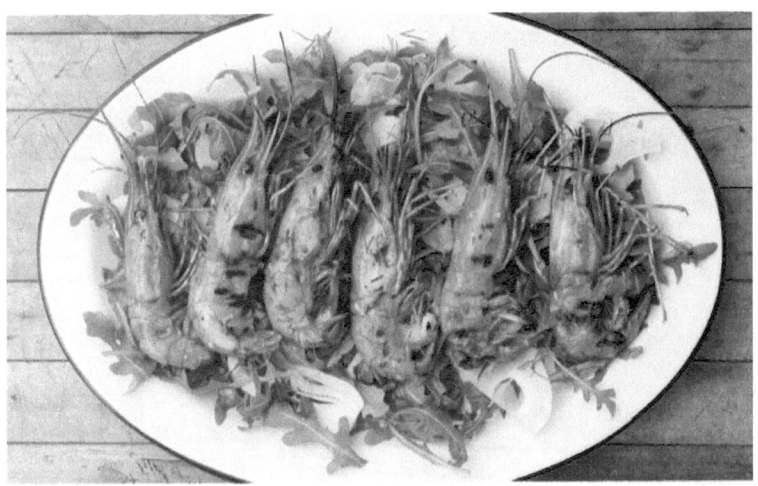

Craving for some sea food? Why not prepare this delicious meal.

Cooking Time: 30 minutes

Serving Size: 1-2

List of Ingredients:

- A pack of de-veined shrimps,
- 2 tsp. of cauliflower,
- ½ cup of broccoli,
- 1 large sliced and diced onion,
- 2 tsp. of olive oil,
- 1 tsp. of lemon juice,
- ½ tsp. of sea salt.

xxxxxxxxxxxxxxxxxxxxxxxxxxxxxxxxxxxxxxxxxxx

Instructions:

Toss the shrimp along with the ingredients, roast the mix until the shrimp turns pink and veggies turn soft, and serve immediately.

Recipe 27: Banana and Berry Smoothie for The Busy Mum

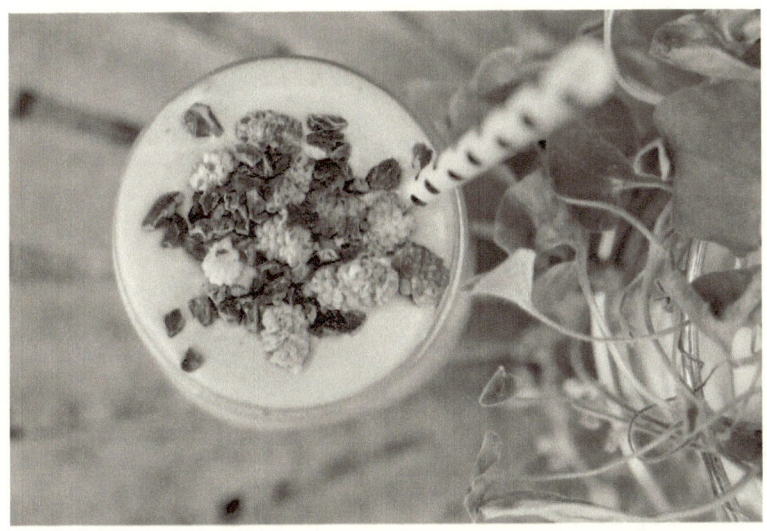

This is a perfect way of starting your day.

Cooking Time: less than 20 minutes

Serving Size: 1-2

List of Ingredients:

- 2 large bananas,
- ½ a cup of frozen mixed berries (including raspberries, blueberries, and blackberries),
- ½ a cup of low fat milk,
- 2 Tbsp. of wheat-germ,
- ½ a cup of low-fat strawberry, and
- 2 tsp. of raw honey.

xxxxxxxxxxxxxxxxxxxxxxxxxxxxxxxxxxxxxxxxxxxxx

Instructions:

Place the ingredients; Banana, berries, wheat-germ, yoghurt, milk and honey inside a jar of blender, blend until perfectly smooth.

Recipe 28: Spaghetti Served with Spinach Meatballs

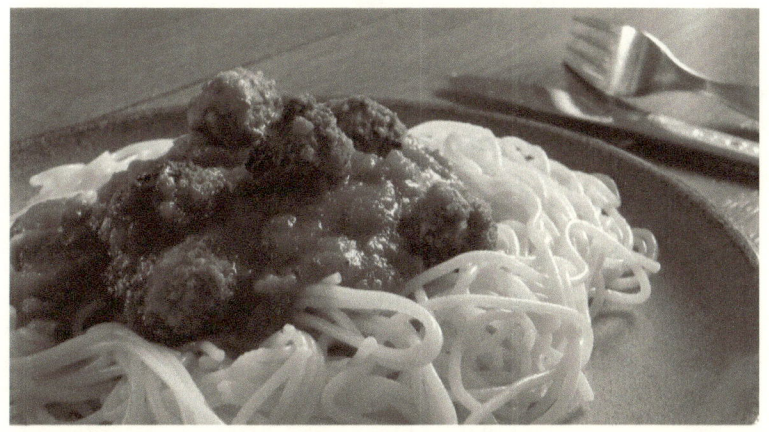

Go organic with this delicious meal. It takes less than 30 minutes.

Cooking Time: 30 minutes

Serving Size: 2

List of Ingredients:

- Sufficient quantities of your favorite spaghetti,
- 2 large tomatoes,
- 2 garlic cloves,
- 2 tsp. of olive oil,
- a handful of pepper flakes,
- A handful of basil,
- ½ cup of ground turkey,
- A cup of your vegetables (kale, spinach)
- A pinch of salt.

xxxxxxxxxxxxxxxxxxxxxxxxxxxxxxxxxxxxxxxxxx

Instructions:

Prepare the spaghetti and toss your ingredients inside. Make the meatballs with some ground turkey, alongside vegetables, then bake in the oven and serve with the spaghetti.

Recipe 29: Mango with Yoghurt Pops

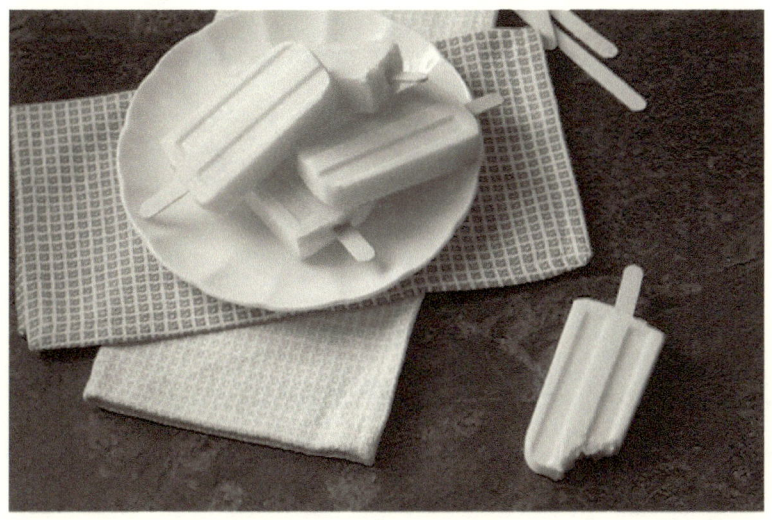

This is a juicy recipe that is very fast to make and packed with healthy nutrients.

Cooking Time: less than 20 minutes

Serving Size: 2-3

List of Ingredients:

- 3 ripe mangoes with the cheeks removed,
- A cup of vanilla yoghurt

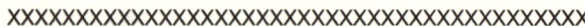

Instructions:

Simply place the mango inside a food processor, and process properly until it becomes smooth. Transfer the mix into a bowl, and then add the vanilla yoghurt. Gently fold the mix of yoghurt and mango until they mix perfectly. Spoon the mi properly.

Recipe 30: The Veggie Pizza

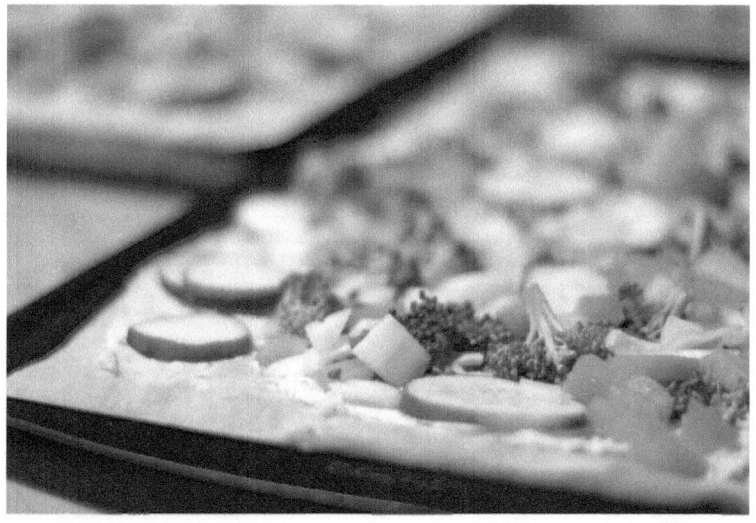

Another wonderful snack for your cravings.

Cooking Time: less than 30 minutes

Serving Size: 4-6

List of Ingredients:

- 2 cups of layer wilted spinach,
- 2 tsp. of fresh basil,
- 1 large sliced caramelized onion,
- 1/3 cup of fire-roasted peppers,
- ½ of cubed chicken,
- ½ cup of whole wheat, and
- 2 tsp. of parmesan.

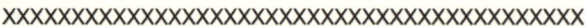

xxxxxxxxxxxxxxxxxxxxxxxxxxxxxxxxxxxxxxxxxxxx

Instructions:

Layer all the ingredients on the wheat pizza, and spray the parmesan. Bake in the oven for about 10 minutes, slice into pieces and serve.

Recipe 31: The Blueberry Pie Protein-Power Smoothie

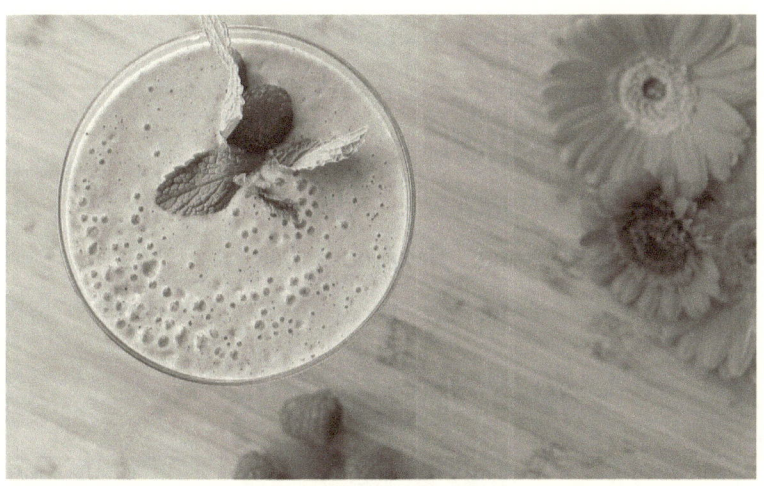

This recipe is ideal for those who want extra antioxidants, fiber, protein and essential minerals such as sodium, in abundance. It provides a total of 216 calories, 14g of protein, 33g of carbs, 4g of fiber, and 115mg of sodium.

Serving Size: 7-10 cups

Cooking Time: less than 15 minutes

List of Ingredients:

- ½ cup of skimmed milk
- a cup of plain fat-free yoghurt
- 2 cups of frozen fresh blueberries
- ½ cup of cooked diced beets
- 1/3 cup of quick oats
- ¼ cup of unflavored vanilla
- ¼ cup of ground flaxseeds
- 2 Tbsp. of blueberry preserves.

xxxxxxxxxxxxxxxxxxxxxxxxxxxxxxxxxxxxxxxxxxx

Instructions: Blend all the ingredients in a juicer or food processor until perfectly smooth.

Recipe 32: Greek Yoghurt with Berries

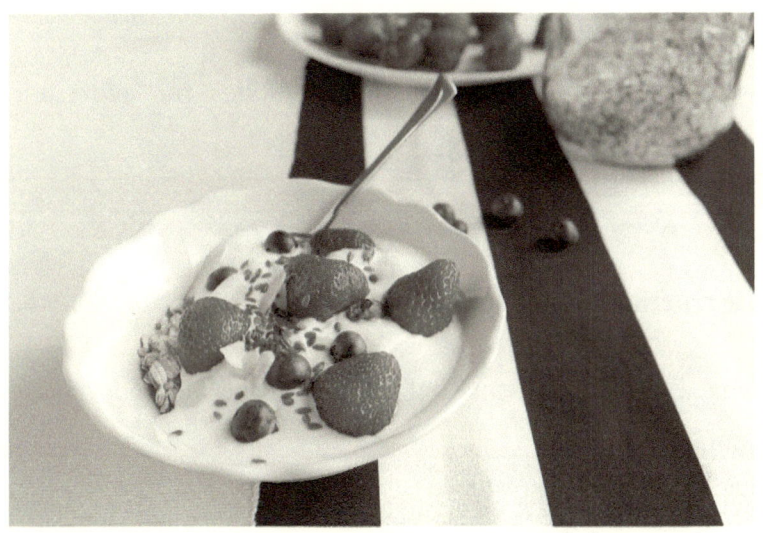

This is a quickie mix for the early morning.

Cooking Time: 10 minutes

Serving Size: 1-2

List of Ingredients:

- A cup of organic plain Greek yoghurt,
- A cup of fresh berries,
- 3 tsp. of vanilla and cinnamon.
- a handful of fresh sliced almonds can add some crunch to the mix.

xxxxxxxxxxxxxxxxxxxxxxxxxxxxxxxxxxxxxxxxxxx

Instructions:

Mix all the ingredients before adding the almonds. Serve immediately.

Recipe 33: The Watercress with Avocado and Tangerine (Evergreen Salad)

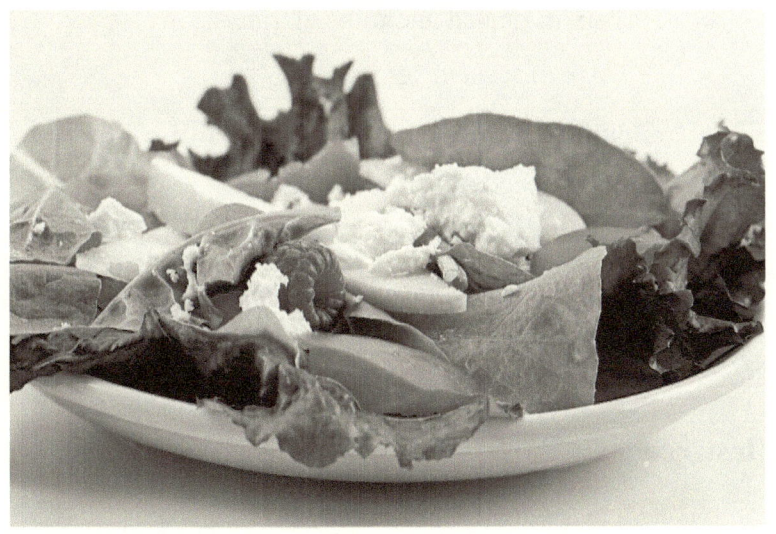

If you need something with some peppery Asian flavours, then this is what you should go for in your Pregnancy Cookbook.

Cooking Time: 30 minutes

Serving Size: 4-6 plates

List of Ingredients:

- 3 Tbsp. of seasoned rice vinegar,
- 3 Tbsp. of chopped shallots,
- 2 Tbsp. of vegetable oil,
- 2 Tbsp. of peeled and minced ginger,
- ½ Tbsp. of toasted sesame oil,
- 2 bunches of trimmed watercress sprigs,
- a cup of sliced mushrooms,
- 4 peeled tangerines 9sliced into halves),
- a large ripe avocado cut into halves.

xxxxxxxxxxxxxxxxxxxxxxxxxxxxxxxxxxxxxxxxxx

Instructions:

Step 1: whisk together the ingredients- shallots, and mushrooms, inside a large bowl and add half of the dressings.

Step 2: Spread the salad on a medium platter, and tuck the tangerine slices with the avocados inside the watercress sprigs, ten drizzle the remaining dressings over the salad.

Step 3: Serve immediately.

Recipe 34: The Nutritious Spinach Smoothie

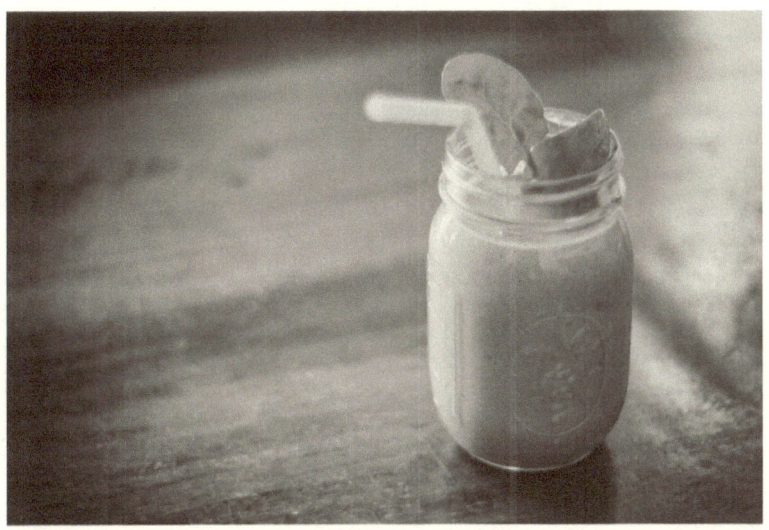

Spinach provides antioxidants that strengthen the immunity of the baby, likewise it comes with essential vitamins and minerals. It is also a cure for morning sicknesses associated with pregnancies

Cooking Time: 15-20 minutes

Serving Size: 1-2

List of Ingredients:

- ½ cup of plain non-fat Greek yoghurt,
- A cup of frozen fruit (this will cover the taste and flavour of spinach),
- ½ cup of sliced spinach,
- 2 Tbsp. of chia seeds,
- ½ a small cup of water.

xxxxxxxxxxxxxxxxxxxxxxxxxxxxxxxxxxxxxxxxxxxxx

Instructions:

Mix all ingredients in the blender and blend properly until smooth. Serve immediately.

Recipe 35: The Quick Egg Salad Recipe (Breakfast)

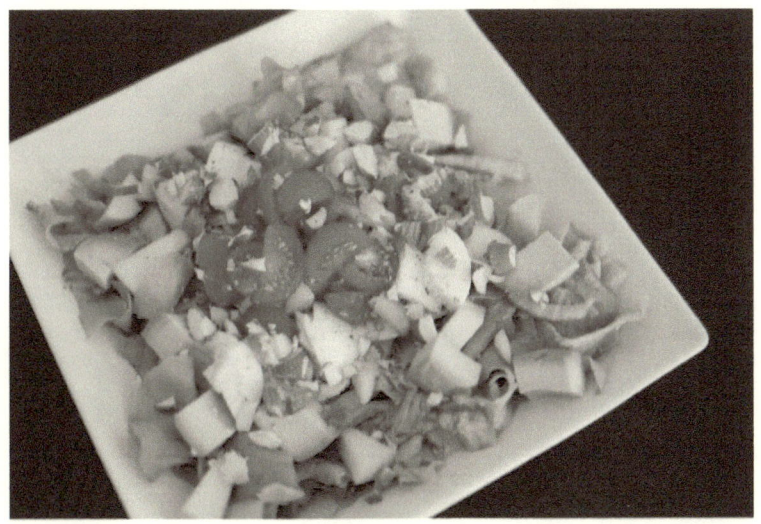

If you are too busy to prepare a large meal, this is what you should go for.

Cooking Time: 20 minutes

Serving Size: 2-3

List of Ingredients:

- 2-3 large eggs,
- a bowl of fresh fruits and vegetable salad
- chopped and diced appropriately
- ½ cup of Greek yoghurt.

xxxxxxxxxxxxxxxxxxxxxxxxxxxxxxxxxxxxxxxxxxxxxxxx

Instructions:

Simply scramble the eggs and prepare over medium heat then serve immediately with the salad and yoghurt.

About the Author

Heston Brown is an accomplished chef and successful e-book author from Palo Alto California. After studying cooking at The New England Culinary Institute, Heston stopped briefly in Chicago where he was offered head chef at some of the city's most prestigious restaurants. Brown decide that he missed the rolling hills and sunny weather of California and moved back to his home state to open up his own catering company and give private cooking classes.

Heston lives in California with his beautiful wife of 18 years and his two daughters who also have aspirations to follow in their father's footsteps and pursue careers in the culinary arts. Brown is well known for his delicious fish and chicken dishes and teaches these recipes as well as many others to his students.

When Heston gave up his successful chef position in Chicago and moved back to California, a friend suggested he use the internet to share his recipes with the world and so he did! To date, Heston Brown has written over 1000 e-books that contain recipes, cooking tips, business strategies for catering companies and a self-help book he wrote from personal experience.

He claims his wife has been his inspiration throughout many of his endeavours and continues to be his partner in business as well as life. His greatest joy is having all three women in his life in the kitchen with him cooking their favourite meal while his favourite jazz music plays in the background.

Author's Afterthoughts

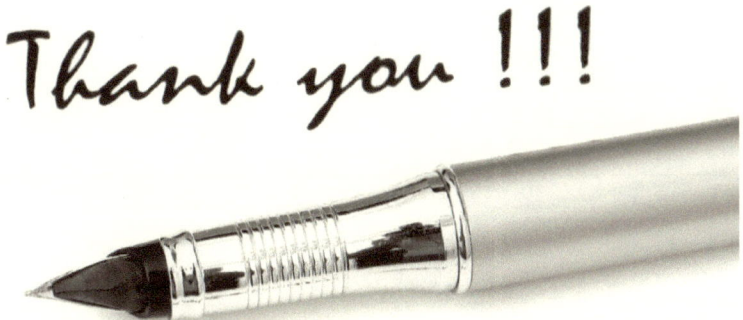

Thank you to all the readers who invested time and money into my book! I cherish every one of you and hope you took the same pleasure in reading it as I did in writing it.

Out of all of the books out there, you chose mine and for that I am truly grateful. It makes the effort worth it when I know my readers are enjoying my work from beginning to end.

Please take a few minutes to write an Amazon review so that others can benefit from your opinions and insight. Your review will help countless other readers make an informed choice

Thank you so much,

Heston Brown

www.ingramcontent.com/pod-product-compliance
Lightning Source LLC
Chambersburg PA
CBHW021231280526
45784CB00005B/2052